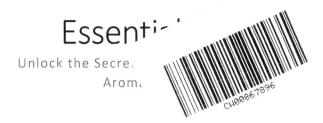

Essenti-'

Unlock the Secre.

Arom.

Emily V. Ste...ıauser

Table of Contents

Acknowledgements

I would like to thank my wonderful Mom and Dad who instilled in me the love to help people live happier and healthier lives.

And to my husband, Paul, who puts up with me researching and writing at the strangest hours.

Essential Oils

Essential oils are oils that are extracted from the flowers, leaves, fruits, peel, seeds, woods, bark, roots, and other natural materials. There are thousands of different kinds of essential oils, and each has unique properties and characteristics. They are highly volatile so they are easily absorbed by the skin. So one wants to take care in the use of them.

Many body care products contain essential oils that they use for their therapeutic properties, and not just for their scent. There are many essential oils that are an effective treatment for a number of different skin conditions. They are extremely concentrated and powerful. They can be regenerative both in physical and emotional ways, making you feel healthy and stronger. The benefits cannot be understated, essential oils can have a dramatic impact on how you look and feel.

This book will explore the various ways that one can use essential oils. I will also present the best oils to use in each specific situation, both from research and personal experience. Sections will focus on the using essential oils to treat, heal, and rejuvenate one's skin. We will also explore how to use essential oils to thicken one's hair, promote faster hair re-growth, and how to deal with hair loss.

Essential oils are often used therapeutically, and I will talk about the medicinal uses of essential oils. I will not only focus on physical application of the oils, but also on aromatherapy and the benefits it provides.

One of my favorite uses of essential oils is using them to deal with headaches, including migraines. They also prove efficacious for first aid, particularly in the reduction of swelling and the healing of bruises. I will also present information on how you can use essential oils to sharpen your mental focus, improve your concentration, and enhance your overall memory.

I am excited that you have joined me on this journey through the essential oils. I hope they bring you a long lifetime of improved health and comfort.

Essential Oils for Skin Treatment

Many skin conditions are preventable if you use essential oils as a daily moisturizer. For instance, dry skin can be prevented by using natural body care products which don't strip your skin of natural oils. Using essential oils can prevent skin problems before they happen.

The best essential oils for normal skin are lavender, rose, rosemary, and rosewood. These oils are for general skin care. The best essential oils to help with dry skin are carrot seeds, cedarwood, clary, jasmine, and oranges. The best essential oils for acne are tea tree, grapefruit, mints, and basil. It is best to apply these oils to your skin at night, so that they are allowed to work over a period of hours.

One of the most popular essential oils for skin care is lavender. Lavender is a highly adaptable oil with soothing properties. It is a small evergreen shrub of the mint family, and is known for its narrow leaves and light purple flowers. It has been widely used in perfume and medicine since ancient times. It is known for being able to relax the mind and body.

Lavender also reduces inflammation and aids in healing. As I mentioned above, it is one of the best oils for normal skin. It can be applied to the skin as a daily natural moisturizer, or it can be used to speed up the healing process of small wounds such as insect bites.

Essential oils can also be used for a number of other skin conditions. Some of which are itchy skin, wrinkles, scars, puffiness, or infections. More often than not essential oils work just as good, if not better than products contain chemicals, and they don't harm your skin in any way.

Essential oils are a great way to make your skin healthier, and using them regularly can prevent future skin problems. They also can be a great natural cure for any existing skin problems you may already have.

Essential Oils for Hair Treatment and Regrowth

Chemicals. Most of us put so many of them in our hair, in the form of shampoo, conditioner, and styling products. This, of course, can have a detrimental effect on the state of our hair. Essential oils can give you beautiful hair that will be incredibly healthy.

One of the benefits of essential oils is that it promotes faster hair growth. Not only do the essential oils clean your hair, they are able to stimulate the circulation in your scalp, resulting in quicker hair growth. Essential oils like rosemary, lavender, thyme, grapefruit, and sage are great for promoting hair growth. As always, you need to experiment to find the oil that works best for you. Also, remember to try various amounts, since sometimes one can see greater results with less oil added.

This ability to give you thicker hair also helps with dealing with any hair loss problems. Strengthening the circulation in the scalp keeps the hair stronger and more resilient, giving you luscious, thick hair. If you feel you are losing too much of your hair, try essential oils like lavender, sage, cypress, rosemary, and lemon. All of these work extremely well for stunting hair loss, while also promoting hair growth.

Another wonderful effect of these essential oils is how they can help you curb dandruff. I've found that not all of the oils work for everyone since dandruff seems to be specific and particular, so experiment with the various oils to see which one works best for you.

As a starting point for hair care, I recommend using lavender or rosemary, and then branch out from there if necessary. You may also notice that an oil may become less effective the longer you use it—I have discovered this problem—so never be afraid to try something new if you are seeing less of an effect on your hair.

Essential Oils as Medicine

One kind of alternative remedy that is commonly used is Essential Oils. Essential oils are known as "essential" because they capture the "essence" of the plant. Unlike oils such as cooking oils, these oils are less fixed and evaporate easily. They also usually have more pleasant aromas.

Although you probably don't realize it, you've been using essential oils your whole life. You've used them in soaps, perfumes, beauty products, and most products that contain natural scents. Essential oils also can be used medically in many different ways.

First there is inhalation therapy. This method is also known as "aromatherapy". A user of the essential oils will inhale the oils by either placing a few drops in a bowl of steaming filtered water, or many people use a diffuser to spread the aroma throughout their room. This method can help relax the user, and help relieve them of any pain, anxiety, or stress they may have. Aromatherapy overall makes the user feel more calm and relaxed.

Second there is topical application. Using essential oils by direct application is a popular method of use. The oil could be used during a massage, or a user could directly place it on their skin to relieve pain on a rash or muscle. Before using an essential oil in this method, you should always test for allergic reactions. Even though the chemical compounds in these types of oils are natural, they could have a negative effect on your body. One example of this is poison ivy.

Third there is Ingestion. Direct ingestion with most essential oils cause a negative effect on the body. Unless you are told by a specialist to do so, this method should only be used with caution. You could consider a tea made with the herb as an alternative if you don't want to inhale the oil or place it on your skin. Although this is a safe mode of internal use, the effect will not be as strong as the other methods mentioned above.

Essential oils have been used as medical treatment since ancient times, and are commonly used all over the world even today. They can be a great natural alternative to many drugs such as anxiety pills or aspirin. They do not replace most medicine though, for they cannot cure any major diseases or intense pain.

It is important to consult a doctor or specialist before using any type of essential oils. It is important to know if they could have a negative effect on your body. It is also wise to ask a doctor about use if you are taking any type of other medication, for the use of both treatments together could also cause a negative effect on your body.

About Using Essential Oils in Aromatherapy

Essential oils have been in use for over six thousand years. Many ancient civilizations documented the use of them in perfumes and drugs. Essential oils were also commonly used in ancient times for spiritual, therapeutic, and even hygienic purposes. For instance, the use of lavender dates back all the way to 500 BC. It was used in ancient times for a form of spiritual healing by the Egyptians and the people of Arabia.

Aromatherapy is the practice of using easily evaporated essential oils from various types of plants to help your health and well-being. Whether they are inhaled or applied to the skin, essential oils are quickly gaining a lot of attention as a natural, alternative treatment for many health problems such as infections, stress, headaches, anxiety, and other forms of health issues.

Aromatherapists apply essential oils to the skin during aromatherapy massages, but the oils also can be released into the air to provide a pleasant, relaxing smell. The oils can be inhaled, or rubbed onto the skin, but they should not be consumed in any way. You should never take essential oils by mouth unless you have specific instruction to do so by a trained specialist.

Fragrances in essential oils activate various nerves in the nose. The nerves then send signals to the part of the brain that is responsible for controlling memory and emotion. The type of essential oil used could result in the body becoming calm and relaxed.

The sense of smell is one of the most powerful senses. Humans can distinguish more than 10,000 unique scents. Along with providing appealing smells, Aromatherapy can help ease a variety of different types of pains. It can be used to ease headaches, body pains, and injuries. Aromatherapy also has several mental health benefits such as stress relief, mood enhancement, anxiety relief, boost of the immune system, and it even can help with depression.

Aromatherapy can be a great, natural health treatment in a wide range of situations. It's definitely not a replacement for prescription medications, because it doesn't cure any major illnesses, although it can relieve discomforts caused by them without interfering with the effects of your normal medication.

Make sure you consult your doctor if you are going to use an alternative therapy, or if you are thinking about combining any form of alternative therapy with your conventional medical treatment, for it may not be safe to combine your medical treatment with any kind of alternative aromatherapy.

Essential Oils for Headaches

One of my favorite uses for essential oils is for headaches. I have found them incredibly effective in either eliminating or greatly minimizing the pain of the headache.

You can either use the essential oils in proper amounts on your skin or you can smell the oils through aromatherapy. Both are very effective, though you may want to experiment with the placement if you decide to apply it directly to your skin. Always follow the directions for applying the proper amount. Places on my skin that I have tried with good effect is on my forehead, my temples, and the top of my neck.

My favorite essential oils for dealing with headaches is peppermint oil and rosemary oil, both which work wonders for me. Basil and lavender also have proven quite effective for me. All of these can work for various types of headaches including migraines.

I have discovered that if your headache gives you a case of nausea that it is best to try smelling the essential oil first. If it upsets your stomach further, it is a good idea not to place the oil on your skin. There is no reason to make yourself feel worse.

Essential Oils for First Aid

Another fantastic use for essential oils is to use them for first aid. Some are incredibly effective in reducing swelling and even helping with bruises. You can also use it to clean cuts and deal with any irritations of the skin. If you plan on cleaning cuts with essential oils, make certain to get a recommendation from your medical provider. Improper use could cause greater irritation.

One of the best general first aid oils is therapeutic level lavender which is extremely versatile. Apply the proper dosage on the area that is inflamed or hurt. Helichrysum is another great essential oil to help prevent inflammation and bruising, since it has the ability to get deep inside the tissue and into the blood stream. Often it is suggested to use helichrysum if the swelling is more severe. For the best results with any essential oil make certain to add a cold compress to your first aid routine to help with the swelling.

I have found that rosehip seed works well for not only dealing with irritation, but also in tackling scarring and wrinkles. For dealing with scarring, rosehip seed needs to be applied once the stitches have been removed. This can help minimize any potential scarring.

Essential Oils for Increasing Brain Power

I swear by the fact that using specific essential oils in aromatherapy has sharpened my mental focus, allowing me to think much clearer, remember much better, and generally feel more alert.

The best essential oils to help with mental acuity are rosemary, peppermint, and basil. One of my morning routines is to smell peppermint to help me wake up. I find it works incredibly well to dismiss the cobwebby feeling I have early in the morning. In fact, I have found it to be more effective than coffee in really sharpening my mind and making me alert in the morning.

Another application is to find a mixture that works well in enhancing your concentration and focus and using it as a perfume to help you throughout your day.

One Last Thing

I hope you have enjoyed this journey through the essential oils as much as I have enjoyed being your guide. Essential oils offer a new world of possibilities if one is patient in exploring and experimenting with them. If you have any questions, make certain to contact your medical provider first. Essential oils are wonderful, but improper use can cause possible discomfort or irritation.

Thank you once again, and good luck!

BONUS: Health Uses of Coconut Oil

Coconut oil is an edible oil with lots of healthy benefits. With an exotic flavor and disease prevention properties it is a fruit with maximum benefits. There are numerous health benefits of coconut. Some of them have been briefly presented for you below:

- Stress decliner: Our busy schedules, the hustles-bustles lead us having a huge amount of stress. Coconut oil massage in such cases, works wonders by relieving us from the stress. The extremely soothing natural aroma of the coconut lowers the stress level and helps us to stay relieved.

- Healthy skin: Healthy skin is something we all strive for. Coconut oil works as a perfect moisturizer for every kind of skins majorly dry and aging skin. The fat of coconut reduces wrinkles without any side effects. Skin problems like psoriasis, dermatitis and eczema can also be treated with the help of coconut oil.

- Healthy, shiny hair: Coconut is the best conditioner for your hair you can opt for. It moisturizes your hair, prevents it from dandruff, supplies essential nutrition in a natural manner unlike the chemical filled conditioners.

- Fit and fine healthy body: Coconut oil has been found very helpful to stimulate your metabolism, improve your thyroid function and increase your energy levels. Coconut oil is indeed the world's only natural low calorie fat which will with its useful traits help you reduce your unwanted fat in an effective manner.

- Antiseptic: Coconut oil also works as an antiseptic. When we apply its oil in cuts and scrapes it forms a thin chemical layer which protects it from outside dust, harmful bacteria and virus. Along with that it also speeds up the healing process by repairing the damaged tissues.

- Digestion: Coconut oil enhances the digesting capability of a person. The saturated fats in the coconut oil carry anti-bacterial properties that help to control parasites and fungi, the prominent causes of indigestion. Not only that the oil also aids in the proper absorption of the vitamins, minerals and amino acids which make you more healthy and strong.

- Increases immune power: Coconut oil enhances the poor immune system and frees your body from frequent attacks of diseases like thyroid, cardio vascular diseases, obesity, cancer and HIV.

- Promotes weight loss: Coconut oil also serves you by letting you lose your weight in a speedy way. It helps to gain a fit slim body.

Coconut oil no doubt has lots of healthy benefits. It helps you solving acne problems, reducing back pain and sore muscles, reducing migraine problems and many more. So, use it to gain the maximum amount of benefits without any side effects.

Preview of "Cellulite Reduction: The Ultimate Guide on How to Get Rid of Cellulite" by Emily V. Steinhauser

What is cellulite in the first place?

As mentioned, cellulite is normal fat or may also be additional fat that is found underneath the connective layers of the skin. The unsightly lines and furrows on the skin develop as the fat pushes against the skin.

Cellulite is more common in women than in men simply because females have more fat tissue compared to their male counterparts. This is because of the difference of fat distribution in a woman's body compared to men. Cellulite may also be present no matter what body type you are which means even thin people have it. Finally, having cellulite does not mean that you are fat it's just that your body is more prone to develop it than other people.

Interesting cellulite facts:

If your parents and other family members have cellulite there is a huge possibility that you will also develop cellulite too.

There are so many reasons why a person develops cellulite, in women; hormones may play a huge role.

You can hardly see cellulite in people with dark skin color but it is still there.

Liposuction is one of the oldest but still effective ways to remove fatty layers on skin however the American Academy of Dermatology cautions about liposuction. They say that it only worsen the appearance of cellulite since the procedure may only create additional depressions on skin.

The best way to remove cellulite is careful planning. This involves a combination of the right diet, exercise, lifestyle changes and the use of effective treatments.

Prevention may help reduce the development of cellulite and prevention also includes diet, exercise and lifestyle changes.

Your dermatologist and your doctor are the best sources of information regarding the removal of cellulite.

What are the signs of cellulite?

First of all you need to spot cellulite to be able to plan how to get rid of it. The common places that you can find cellulite are parts of the body where excess fat usually deposit. Thus you may find cellulite on the thighs, the hips, buttocks, upper arms, on the midsection and sometimes on the neck area. Skin may appear

- Dimpled and uneven

- With obvious irregular marks on the surface of the skin

- There is discoloration along the area especially when viewed under natural light

Knowing the signs of cellulite will help people develop the ideal cellulite removal plan. Since cellulite may be reduced, if not removed, with the use of exercise, the ideal exercise regimen to tone the area with cellulite may be done.

I hope you enjoyed this free preview of "Cellulite Reduction: The Ultimate Guide on How to Get Rid of Cellulite" by Emily V. Steinhauser.

Click here to check out the rest of Cellulite Reduction by Emily V. Steinhauser on Amazon.com.

Or go to: http://amzn.to/1fUyAVj

Preview of "Speed Reading Training" by Warren R. Sullivan

Chapter 1

How people usually read

Before you begin to improve your reading speed, you should first find out how you really read or how you understand texts. Naturally people use the following strategies to be able to read different texts and sentences in their everyday life. How a person reads may be according to how he needs to read in the first place; this is called reading according to purpose.

For instance, a person who reads the morning paper could have a reading skill that is different from a person that is reading an instruction on how to operate a machine. Basically how we read is what we are. Lawyers tend to read books and reports more diligently compared to someone that only reads for leisure.

In most cases, the way people read may be classified according to the following:

Skimming

Skimming is reading that looks only for the general idea of a reading material. It is just like what the word is, you are just reading parts of the story, article or report in a generalized manner. Most people use skimming reading when the article, story or selection that they are to read is quite long and the topic may not be appealing to them.

Students use skimming when they cram; it's like mediocre reading since you claim you have read the text but in reality you have read only a portion of it. Skimming may speed up reading but it may not work all the time in understanding a text.

Scanning

Scanning may be similar to skimming but you are mainly looking at specific facts that are in a text. You are not reading an entire text at all but instead you are only reading specific information. This may work for informative reading material but not for fictional reading or literature. It works great in reading instructions and how-to articles since you do not waste time reading introductions but you would rather get on with more important part of your text.

Intensive or functional

Functional reading is all about reading with a deeper purpose and that is to understand the reading material to acquire newer and more complex skills and new knowledge. Although this technique is ideal in retaining learning for a long period of time it may require time to do and thus could be time consuming.

Extensive or recreational

Recreational or extensive reading is simply relaxed reading. This kind of reading is done by book lovers as they read a book that they intend for leisure purposes. You read in a recreational manner and may at the same time let your imagination take flight as you imagine yourself being a character or an element in the story. A person that does extensive reading may read in whatever pace he is comfortable with; there is no rush but if he can read using speed reading techniques he may be able to finish as many stories or books as he can.

You may adapt a variety of reading types and may use one for a particular activity. However, by using speed reading techniques you can double or triple the amount of topics, articles and paragraphs that you can read and understand in one sitting! And remember that the more you read the more you will learn so technically you will be able to learn a lot when you adapt speed reading in your everyday activities.

I hope you enjoyed the free preview of "Speed Reading Training" by Warren R. Sullivan.

Click here to check out the rest of Speed Reading Training on Amazon.

Or go to: http://amzn.to/1jjip2P

Preview of "Kindle Publishing Secrets Revealed" by James Chen

Learn to Make Money with Kindle Books

Passive income. We all want to make it. And publishing books on Amazon Kindle is a great way to do it. Imagine your books earning money 24 hours a day, 365 days a year on autopilot, leaving you the time to do whatever you desire. Sounds like a wonderful life, right?

It can be, and the first step is publishing your book. This book will guide you step by step through the process, from initial research to how to market your book.

Don't think you are a very good writer? I will show you how outsource your ideas to other writers who will write the books for you. All you need to do is publish them. And collect the checks.

I will also divulge a secret niche which sees extraordinary sales and searches on Amazon. There are very few writers taking advantage of this trick, and those who have are seeing their books in the bestseller lists. The best part: this niche only requires the books be between 15 to 30 pages in length. Short books, huge rewards.

Learn to take advantage of Amazon's enormous customer base, publishing books that will be searched for, found, and purchased. Learn to get your books to stand out from the millions of other ones already available in the Kindle store. It is simple: if people cannot find your books, they will not buy them. Learn how to be found.

The #1 Rule of Kindle Marketing

The rule is simple: find a process that makes money. And repeat it. Over and over again. This rule is particularly effective in terms of Kindle publishing. You publish your book, market it, let it make money, and do the entire process again.

Too many writers concentrate on one book. They invest all of their energy in making it perfect, trying to build up and audience, instead of writing additional books. Understand that having one book found within millions of books requires a whole lot of luck. But if you have two books, your odds increase. Think of each book as a lottery ticket, the more you have, the more likely you will have one hit the jackpot. Your goal should not be to have one book in the Kindle store, but hundreds. Don't imagine yourself as a writer, but as a publisher. And act accordingly.

Authors often focus on the visible success stories on Amazon, on the fiction writers who have sold hundreds of thousands of books. This is an incredibly small group, and their success is hard to replicate, because it was brought about by luck. You will most likely never get this lucky, so you need to create your own success. That means publishing a lot of books.

The people making money in the system are those who publish hundreds of books under different pen names. These books are often outsourced to a group of writers, as are the formatting and cover creation. This book encourages you to embrace the second method and act like a publisher, producing and selling as much content as you can.

Remember the more you publish, the larger your slice of the pie will be.

I hope you enjoyed the free preview of "Kindle Publishing Secrets Revealed" by James Chen.

Click here to check out the rest of Kindle Publishing Secrets Revealed on Amazon.

Or go to: http://www.amazon.com/dp/B00K5I3MC0/

Other Books Available From Gamma Mouse Media

Below you will find other popular Amazon bestsellers from Gamma Mouse Media. Simply click on the links to check them out.

Forex Indicators – Warren R. Sullivan

Kindle Publishing Secrets Revealed – James Chen

Procrastination – Warren R. Sullivan

Brain Training Boot Camp – Warren R. Sullivan

Knee Pain Treatment – Emily V. Steinhauser

Marriage Problems – Emily V. Steinhauser

Quiet – Amelia Austin

Lust for Me – Amelia Austin

Cellulite Reduction – Emily V. Steinhauser

The Quick Start Guide to Macarons – Lindsay Stotts

Speed Reading Training – Warren R. Sullivan

Memory Enhancement – Warren R. Sullivan

The Quick Start Guide to Perfect Pancakes – Lindsay Stotts

Compulsive Hoarding – Emily V. Steinhauser

If the links above do not work, you can simply search for these titles on Amazon's website to find them.

9570844R00027

Printed in Great Britain
by Amazon.co.uk, Ltd.,
Marston Gate.